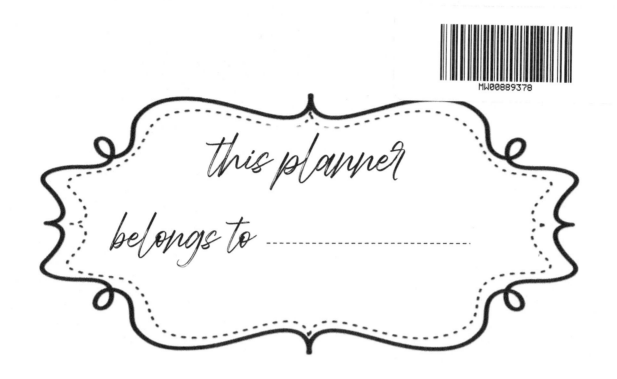

this planner

belongs to ----------------------------------

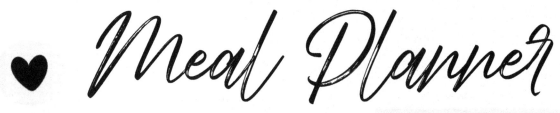# Meal Planner

WEEK NUMBER:

MONDAY

TUESDAY

WEDNESDAY

THURSDAY

FRIDAY

SATURDAY

SUNDAY

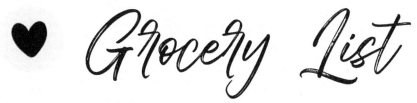

Grocery List

GROCERY BUDGET: _____

PRODUCE

_____
_____
_____
_____
_____
_____

MEAT · POULTRY · FISH

_____
_____
_____
_____
_____

CANNED · FROZEN

_____
_____
_____
_____
_____
_____

BREADS · PASTA · GRAINS

_____
_____
_____
_____
_____

DAIRY · CHEESE · EGGS

_____
_____
_____
_____
_____
_____

SNACKS · BEVERAGES

_____
_____
_____
_____
_____
_____

NON-FOOD ITEMS

_____
_____
_____
_____

notes

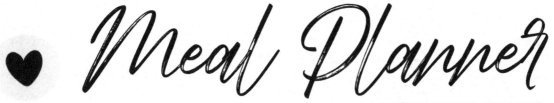# Meal Planner

WEEK NUMBER:

MONDAY

TUESDAY

WEDNESDAY

THURSDAY

FRIDAY

SATURDAY

SUNDAY

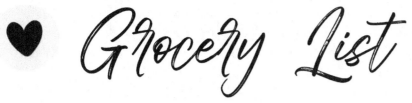

Grocery List

GROCERY BUDGET: _____

PRODUCE

_____
_____
_____
_____
_____
_____

MEAT • POULTRY • FISH

_____
_____
_____
_____
_____
_____

CANNED • FROZEN

_____
_____
_____
_____
_____

BREADS • PASTA • GRAINS

_____
_____
_____
_____
_____

DAIRY • CHEESE • EGGS

_____
_____
_____
_____
_____

SNACKS • BEVERAGES

_____
_____
_____
_____
_____

NON-FOOD ITEMS

_____
_____
_____
_____

notes

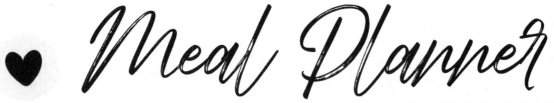

Meal Planner

WEEK NUMBER:

MONDAY

TUESDAY

WEDNESDAY

THURSDAY

FRIDAY

SATURDAY

SUNDAY

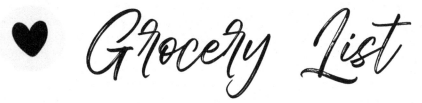

Grocery List

GROCERY BUDGET:

PRODUCE

BREADS · PASTA · GRAINS

MEAT · POULTRY · FISH

DAIRY · CHEESE · EGGS

CANNED · FROZEN

SNACKS · BEVERAGES

NON-FOOD ITEMS

notes

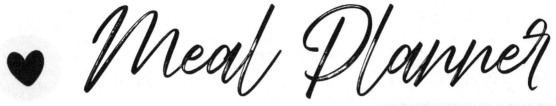

Meal Planner

MONDAY

TUESDAY

WEDNESDAY

THURSDAY

FRIDAY

SATURDAY

SUNDAY

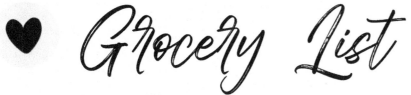

Grocery List

GROCERY BUDGET:

PRODUCE

_____
_____
_____
_____
_____
_____

MEAT · POULTRY · FISH

_____
_____
_____
_____
_____
_____

CANNED · FROZEN

_____
_____
_____
_____
_____
_____

BREADS · PASTA · GRAINS

_____
_____
_____
_____
_____
_____

DAIRY · CHEESE · EGGS

_____
_____
_____
_____
_____
_____

SNACKS · BEVERAGES

_____
_____
_____
_____
_____
_____

NON-FOOD ITEMS

_____
_____
_____
_____

notes

Notes

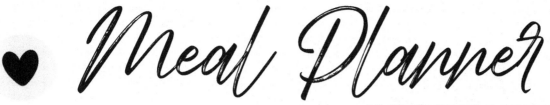

Meal Planner

WEEK NUMBER:

MONDAY

TUESDAY

WEDNESDAY

THURSDAY

FRIDAY

SATURDAY

SUNDAY

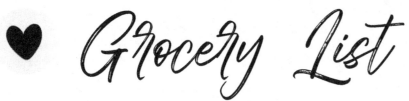

Grocery List

PRODUCE

BREADS • PASTA • GRAINS

_____

_____

_____

_____

_____

MEAT • POULTRY • FISH

DAIRY • CHEESE • EGGS

_____

_____

_____

_____

CANNED • FROZEN

SNACKS • BEVERAGES

_____

_____

_____

_____

notes

NON-FOOD ITEMS

_____

_____

_____

_____

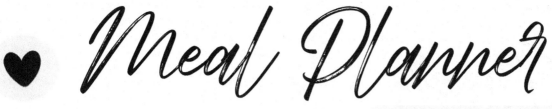

Meal Planner

WEEK NUMBER:

MONDAY

TUESDAY

WEDNESDAY

THURSDAY

FRIDAY

SATURDAY

SUNDAY

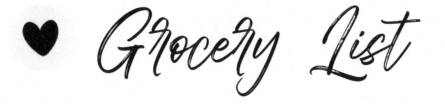

Grocery List

GROCERY BUDGET:

PRODUCE

BREADS • PASTA • GRAINS

MEAT • POULTRY • FISH

DAIRY • CHEESE • EGGS

CANNED • FROZEN

SNACKS • BEVERAGES

NON-FOOD ITEMS

notes

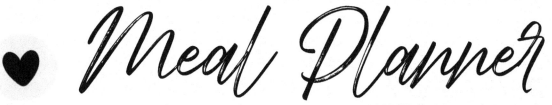

Meal Planner

WEEK NUMBER:

MONDAY

TUESDAY

WEDNESDAY

THURSDAY

FRIDAY

SATURDAY

SUNDAY

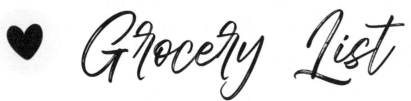

Grocery List

GROCERY BUDGET:

PRODUCE

_____

BREADS • PASTA • GRAINS

_____

_____

_____

_____

_____

_____

_____

_____

_____

_____

_____

_____

DAIRY • CHEESE • EGGS

_____

MEAT • POULTRY • FISH

_____

_____

_____

_____

_____

_____

_____

_____

_____

_____

_____

_____

_____

SNACKS • BEVERAGES

_____

CANNED • FROZEN

_____

_____

_____

_____

_____

_____

_____

_____

_____

_____

_____

NON-FOOD ITEMS

notes

_____

_____

_____

_____

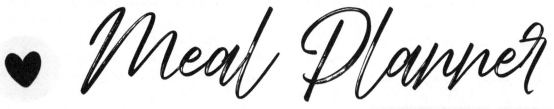

Meal Planner

WEEK NUMBER:

MONDAY

TUESDAY

WEDNESDAY

THURSDAY

FRIDAY

SATURDAY

SUNDAY

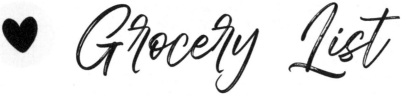

Grocery List

PRODUCE

BREADS • PASTA • GRAINS

DAIRY • CHEESE • EGGS

MEAT • POULTRY • FISH

SNACKS • BEVERAGES

CANNED • FROZEN

NON-FOOD ITEMS

notes

Notes

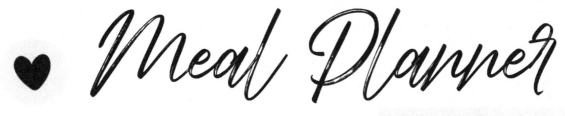# Meal Planner

MONDAY

TUESDAY

WEDNESDAY

THURSDAY

FRIDAY

SATURDAY

SUNDAY

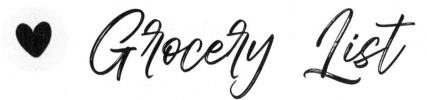

Grocery List

GROCERY BUDGET:

PRODUCE

_____

_____

_____

_____

_____

_____

MEAT • POULTRY • FISH

_____

_____

_____

_____

_____

_____

CANNED • FROZEN

_____

_____

_____

_____

_____

_____

BREADS • PASTA • GRAINS

_____

_____

_____

_____

_____

_____

DAIRY • CHEESE • EGGS

_____

_____

_____

_____

_____

_____

SNACKS • BEVERAGES

_____

_____

_____

_____

_____

_____

NON-FOOD ITEMS

_____

_____

_____

_____

_____

notes

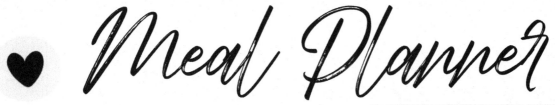# Meal Planner

WEEK NUMBER:

MONDAY

TUESDAY

WEDNESDAY

THURSDAY

FRIDAY

SATURDAY

SUNDAY

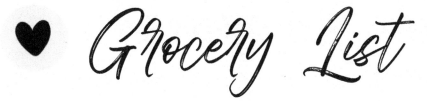

Grocery List

GROCERY BUDGET:

BREADS · PASTA · GRAINS

_____
_____
_____
_____
_____

PRODUCE

_____
_____
_____
_____
_____
_____

DAIRY · CHEESE · EGGS

_____
_____
_____
_____
_____
_____
_____

MEAT · POULTRY · FISH

_____
_____
_____
_____
_____
_____

SNACKS · BEVERAGES

_____
_____
_____
_____
_____
_____
_____

CANNED · FROZEN

_____
_____
_____
_____
_____

NON-FOOD ITEMS

_____
_____
_____
_____
_____

notes

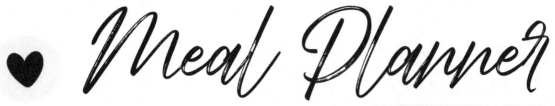

Meal Planner

WEEK NUMBER:

MONDAY

TUESDAY

WEDNESDAY

THURSDAY

FRIDAY

SATURDAY

SUNDAY

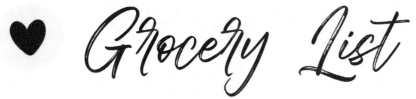

Grocery List

PRODUCE

_____
_____
_____
_____
_____

MEAT · POULTRY · FISH

_____
_____
_____
_____
_____

CANNED · FROZEN

_____
_____
_____
_____
_____

BREADS · PASTA · GRAINS

_____
_____
_____
_____

DAIRY · CHEESE · EGGS

_____
_____
_____
_____
_____

SNACKS · BEVERAGES

_____
_____
_____
_____
_____

NON-FOOD ITEMS

_____
_____
_____
_____

notes

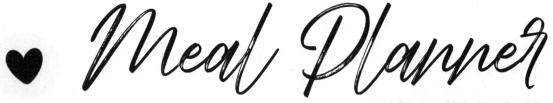

Meal Planner

WEEK NUMBER:

MONDAY

TUESDAY

WEDNESDAY

THURSDAY

FRIDAY

SATURDAY

SUNDAY

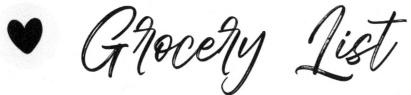

Grocery List

GROCERY BUDGET:

PRODUCE

BREADS · PASTA · GRAINS

MEAT · POULTRY · FISH

DAIRY · CHEESE · EGGS

SNACKS · BEVERAGES

CANNED · FROZEN

NON-FOOD ITEMS

notes

Notes

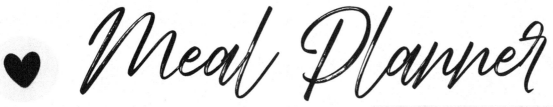

Meal Planner

WEEK NUMBER:

MONDAY

TUESDAY

WEDNESDAY

THURSDAY

FRIDAY

SATURDAY

SUNDAY

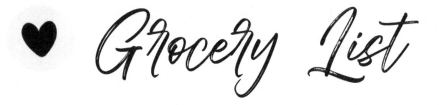

Grocery List

GROCERY BUDGET:

PRODUCE

BREADS · PASTA · GRAINS

MEAT · POULTRY · FISH

DAIRY · CHEESE · EGGS

CANNED · FROZEN

SNACKS · BEVERAGES

NON-FOOD ITEMS

notes

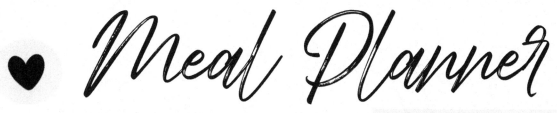# Meal Planner

WEEK NUMBER:

MONDAY

TUESDAY

WEDNESDAY

THURSDAY

FRIDAY

SATURDAY

SUNDAY

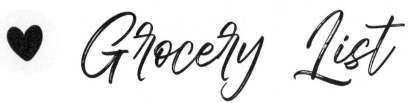

Grocery List

GROCERY BUDGET:

PRODUCE

BREADS · PASTA · GRAINS

MEAT · POULTRY · FISH

DAIRY · CHEESE · EGGS

CANNED · FROZEN

SNACKS · BEVERAGES

NON-FOOD ITEMS

notes

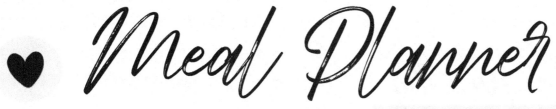

Meal Planner

WEEK NUMBER:

MONDAY

TUESDAY

WEDNESDAY

THURSDAY

FRIDAY

SATURDAY

SUNDAY

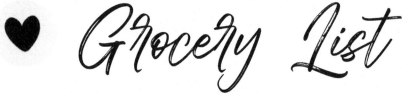

Grocery List

PRODUCE

BREADS · PASTA · GRAINS

DAIRY · CHEESE · EGGS

MEAT · POULTRY · FISH

SNACKS · BEVERAGES

CANNED · FROZEN

NON-FOOD ITEMS

notes

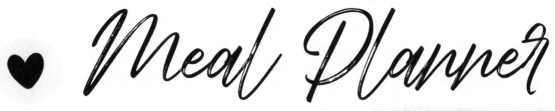

Meal Planner

WEEK NUMBER:

MONDAY

TUESDAY

WEDNESDAY

THURSDAY

FRIDAY

SATURDAY

SUNDAY

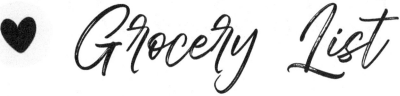

Grocery List

GROCERY BUDGET:

PRODUCE

BREADS · PASTA · GRAINS

MEAT · POULTRY · FISH

DAIRY · CHEESE · EGGS

CANNED · FROZEN

SNACKS · BEVERAGES

NON-FOOD ITEMS

notes

Notes

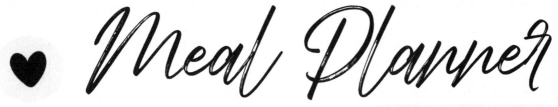 # Meal Planner

WEEK NUMBER:

MONDAY

TUESDAY

WEDNESDAY

THURSDAY

FRIDAY

SATURDAY

SUNDAY

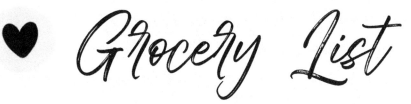

Grocery List

GROCERY BUDGET:

PRODUCE

BREADS • PASTA • GRAINS

MEAT • POULTRY • FISH

DAIRY • CHEESE • EGGS

CANNED • FROZEN

SNACKS • BEVERAGES

NON-FOOD ITEMS

notes

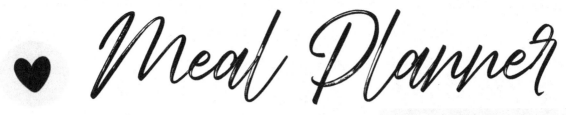

Meal Planner

WEEK NUMBER:

MONDAY

TUESDAY

WEDNESDAY

THURSDAY

FRIDAY

SATURDAY

SUNDAY

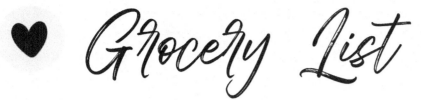

Grocery List

GROCERY BUDGET:

PRODUCE

_____

BREADS · PASTA · GRAINS

_____

MEAT · POULTRY · FISH

DAIRY · CHEESE · EGGS

CANNED · FROZEN

SNACKS · BEVERAGES

NON-FOOD ITEMS

notes

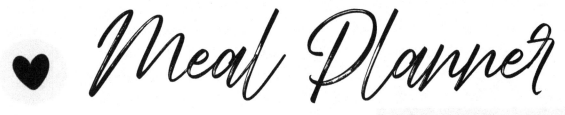

Meal Planner

WEEK NUMBER:

MONDAY

TUESDAY

WEDNESDAY

THURSDAY

FRIDAY

SATURDAY

SUNDAY

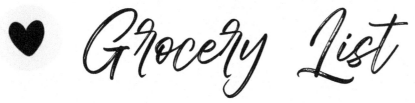

Grocery List

GROCERY BUDGET:

PRODUCE

BREADS · PASTA · GRAINS

MEAT · POULTRY · FISH

DAIRY · CHEESE · EGGS

SNACKS · BEVERAGES

CANNED · FROZEN

NON-FOOD ITEMS

notes

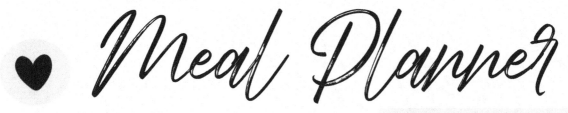

Meal Planner

WEEK NUMBER:

MONDAY

TUESDAY

WEDNESDAY

THURSDAY

FRIDAY

SATURDAY

SUNDAY

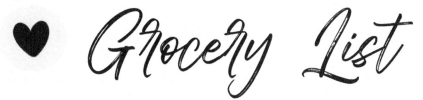

Grocery List

GROCERY BUDGET:

PRODUCE

_____
_____
_____
_____
_____
_____

MEAT · POULTRY · FISH

_____
_____
_____
_____
_____
_____

CANNED · FROZEN

_____
_____
_____
_____
_____
_____

BREADS · PASTA · GRAINS

_____
_____
_____
_____

DAIRY · CHEESE · EGGS

_____
_____
_____
_____
_____

SNACKS · BEVERAGES

_____
_____
_____
_____
_____
_____

NON-FOOD ITEMS

_____
_____
_____
_____

notes

Notes

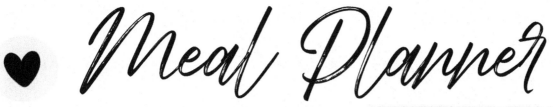

Meal Planner

WEEK NUMBER:

MONDAY

TUESDAY

WEDNESDAY

THURSDAY

FRIDAY

SATURDAY

SUNDAY

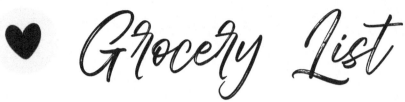

Grocery List

PRODUCE

_____

_____

_____

_____

_____

_____

MEAT · POULTRY · FISH

_____

_____

_____

_____

_____

_____

CANNED · FROZEN

_____

_____

_____

_____

_____

notes

GROCERY BUDGET:

BREADS · PASTA · GRAINS

_____

_____

_____

_____

_____

DAIRY · CHEESE · EGGS

_____

_____

_____

_____

_____

SNACKS · BEVERAGES

_____

_____

_____

_____

_____

NON-FOOD ITEMS

_____

_____

_____

_____

_____

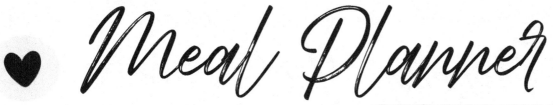

Meal Planner

WEEK NUMBER:

MONDAY

TUESDAY

WEDNESDAY

THURSDAY

FRIDAY

SATURDAY

SUNDAY

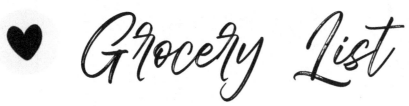

Grocery List

GROCERY BUDGET:

PRODUCE

BREADS · PASTA · GRAINS

MEAT · POULTRY · FISH

DAIRY · CHEESE · EGGS

CANNED · FROZEN

SNACKS · BEVERAGES

NON-FOOD ITEMS

notes

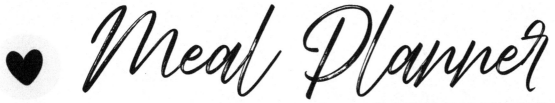

Meal Planner

WEEK NUMBER:

MONDAY

TUESDAY

WEDNESDAY

THURSDAY

FRIDAY

SATURDAY

SUNDAY

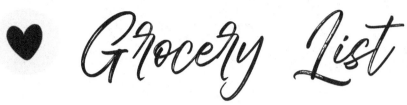

Grocery List

GROCERY BUDGET:

PRODUCE

BREADS • PASTA • GRAINS

MEAT • POULTRY • FISH

DAIRY • CHEESE • EGGS

SNACKS • BEVERAGES

CANNED • FROZEN

NON-FOOD ITEMS

notes

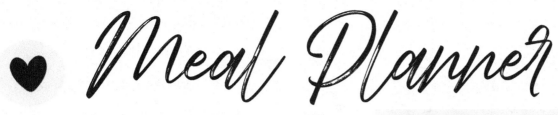

Meal Planner

WEEK NUMBER:

MONDAY

TUESDAY

WEDNESDAY

THURSDAY

FRIDAY

SATURDAY

SUNDAY

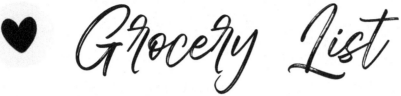

Grocery List

PRODUCE

GROCERY BUDGET:

BREADS · PASTA · GRAINS

MEAT · POULTRY · FISH

DAIRY · CHEESE · EGGS

SNACKS · BEVERAGES

CANNED · FROZEN

NON-FOOD ITEMS

notes

Notes

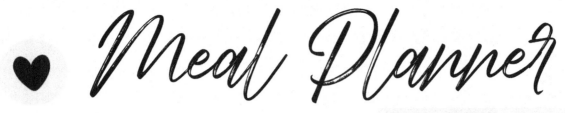 *Meal Planner*

WEEK NUMBER:

MONDAY

TUESDAY

WEDNESDAY

THURSDAY

FRIDAY

SATURDAY

SUNDAY

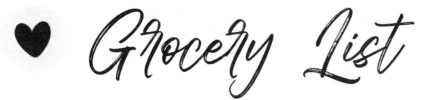

Grocery List

GROCERY BUDGET:

PRODUCE

_____
_____
_____
_____
_____
_____

MEAT · POULTRY · FISH

_____
_____
_____
_____
_____
_____

CANNED · FROZEN

_____
_____
_____
_____
_____
_____

BREADS · PASTA · GRAINS

_____
_____
_____
_____
_____

DAIRY · CHEESE · EGGS

_____
_____
_____
_____
_____
_____

SNACKS · BEVERAGES

_____
_____
_____
_____
_____
_____

NON-FOOD ITEMS

_____
_____
_____
_____

notes

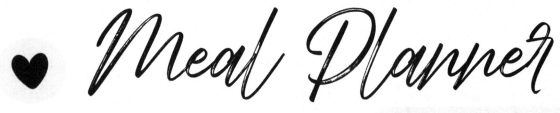

Meal Planner

WEEK NUMBER:

MONDAY

TUESDAY

WEDNESDAY

THURSDAY

FRIDAY

SATURDAY

SUNDAY

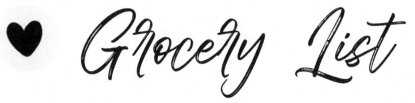

Grocery List

GROCERY BUDGET: _____

PRODUCE

_____

_____

_____

_____

_____

MEAT · POULTRY · FISH

_____

_____

_____

_____

_____

CANNED · FROZEN

_____

_____

_____

_____

_____

BREADS · PASTA · GRAINS

_____

_____

_____

_____

_____

DAIRY · CHEESE · EGGS

_____

_____

_____

_____

_____

SNACKS · BEVERAGES

_____

_____

_____

_____

_____

NON-FOOD ITEMS

_____

_____

_____

_____

notes

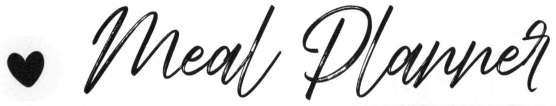 Meal Planner

WEEK NUMBER:

MONDAY

TUESDAY

WEDNESDAY

THURSDAY

FRIDAY

SATURDAY

SUNDAY

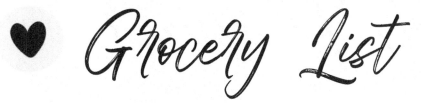

Grocery List

GROCERY BUDGET:

PRODUCE

BREADS · PASTA · GRAINS

MEAT · POULTRY · FISH

DAIRY · CHEESE · EGGS

CANNED · FROZEN

SNACKS · BEVERAGES

NON-FOOD ITEMS

notes

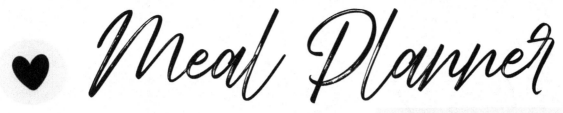

Meal Planner

WEEK NUMBER:

MONDAY

TUESDAY

WEDNESDAY

THURSDAY

FRIDAY

SATURDAY

SUNDAY

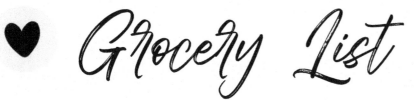

Grocery List

GROCERY BUDGET:

PRODUCE

BREADS · PASTA · GRAINS

MEAT · POULTRY · FISH

DAIRY · CHEESE · EGGS

CANNED · FROZEN

SNACKS · BEVERAGES

NON-FOOD ITEMS

notes

Notes

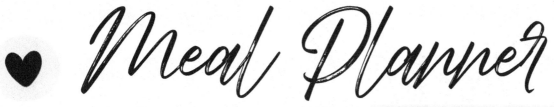

Meal Planner

WEEK NUMBER:

MONDAY

TUESDAY

WEDNESDAY

THURSDAY

FRIDAY

SATURDAY

SUNDAY

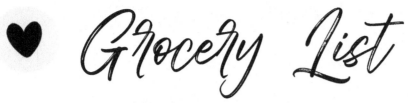

Grocery List

GROCERY BUDGET:

PRODUCE

BREADS · PASTA · GRAINS

MEAT · POULTRY · FISH

DAIRY · CHEESE · EGGS

CANNED · FROZEN

SNACKS · BEVERAGES

NON-FOOD ITEMS

notes

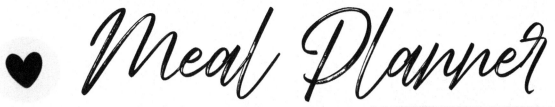

Meal Planner

WEEK NUMBER:

MONDAY

TUESDAY

WEDNESDAY

THURSDAY

FRIDAY

SATURDAY

SUNDAY

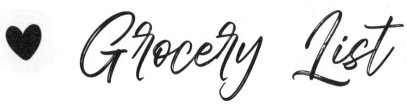

Grocery List

BREADS • PASTA • GRAINS

PRODUCE

DAIRY • CHEESE • EGGS

MEAT • POULTRY • FISH

SNACKS • BEVERAGES

CANNED • FROZEN

NON-FOOD ITEMS

notes

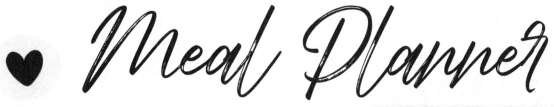

Meal Planner

WEEK NUMBER:

MONDAY

TUESDAY

WEDNESDAY

THURSDAY

FRIDAY

SATURDAY

SUNDAY

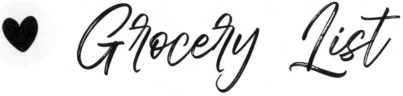

Grocery List

GROCERY BUDGET:

PRODUCE

_____
_____
_____
_____
_____
_____

MEAT · POULTRY · FISH

_____
_____
_____
_____
_____
_____

CANNED · FROZEN

_____
_____
_____
_____
_____

BREADS · PASTA · GRAINS

_____
_____
_____
_____
_____

DAIRY · CHEESE · EGGS

_____
_____
_____
_____
_____

SNACKS · BEVERAGES

_____
_____
_____
_____
_____

NON-FOOD ITEMS

_____
_____
_____
_____

notes

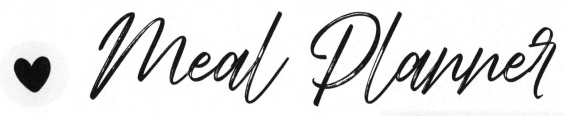

Meal Planner

WEEK NUMBER:

MONDAY

TUESDAY

WEDNESDAY

THURSDAY

FRIDAY

SATURDAY

SUNDAY

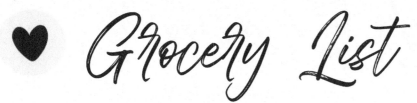

Grocery List

GROCERY BUDGET:

PRODUCE

BREADS · PASTA · GRAINS

DAIRY · CHEESE · EGGS

MEAT · POULTRY · FISH

SNACKS · BEVERAGES

CANNED · FROZEN

NON-FOOD ITEMS

notes

Notes

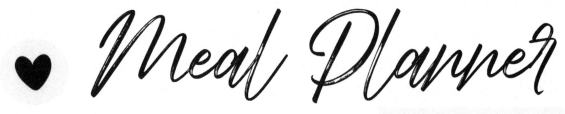

Meal Planner

WEEK NUMBER:

MONDAY

TUESDAY

WEDNESDAY

THURSDAY

FRIDAY

SATURDAY

SUNDAY

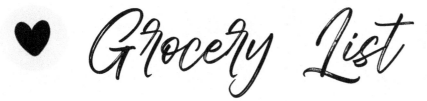

Grocery List

GROCERY BUDGET:

BREADS · PASTA · GRAINS

PRODUCE

MEAT · POULTRY · FISH

DAIRY · CHEESE · EGGS

CANNED · FROZEN

SNACKS · BEVERAGES

NON-FOOD ITEMS

notes

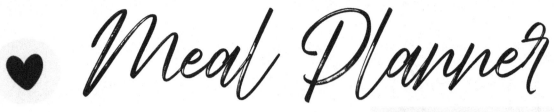

Meal Planner

WEEK NUMBER:

MONDAY

TUESDAY

WEDNESDAY

THURSDAY

FRIDAY

SATURDAY

SUNDAY

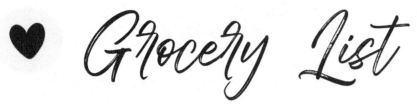

Grocery List

GROCERY BUDGET:

BREADS · PASTA · GRAINS

PRODUCE

MEAT · POULTRY · FISH

DAIRY · CHEESE · EGGS

SNACKS · BEVERAGES

CANNED · FROZEN

NON-FOOD ITEMS

notes

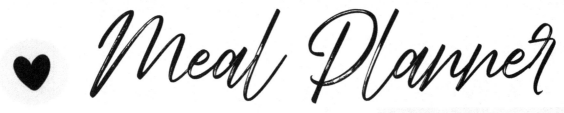

Meal Planner

WEEK NUMBER:

MONDAY

TUESDAY

WEDNESDAY

THURSDAY

FRIDAY

SATURDAY

SUNDAY

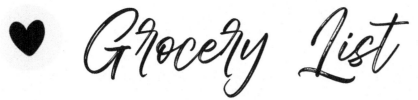

Grocery List

GROCERY BUDGET: _____

PRODUCE

BREADS · PASTA · GRAINS

DAIRY · CHEESE · EGGS

MEAT · POULTRY · FISH

SNACKS · BEVERAGES

CANNED · FROZEN

NON-FOOD ITEMS

notes

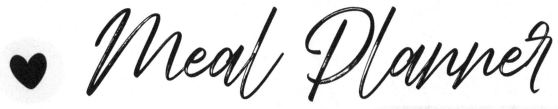

Meal Planner

WEEK NUMBER:

MONDAY

TUESDAY

WEDNESDAY

THURSDAY

FRIDAY

SATURDAY

SUNDAY

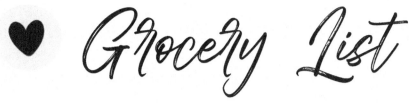

Grocery List

GROCERY BUDGET:

PRODUCE

_____
_____
_____
_____
_____
_____

MEAT · POULTRY · FISH

_____
_____
_____
_____
_____
_____

CANNED · FROZEN

_____
_____
_____
_____
_____
_____

BREADS · PASTA · GRAINS

_____
_____
_____
_____
_____

DAIRY · CHEESE · EGGS

_____
_____
_____
_____
_____

SNACKS · BEVERAGES

_____
_____
_____
_____
_____

NON-FOOD ITEMS

_____
_____
_____
_____

notes

Notes

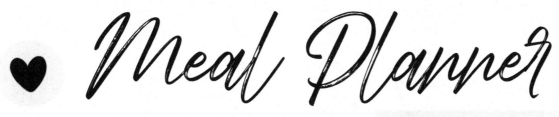

Meal Planner

WEEK NUMBER:

MONDAY

TUESDAY

WEDNESDAY

THURSDAY

FRIDAY

SATURDAY

SUNDAY

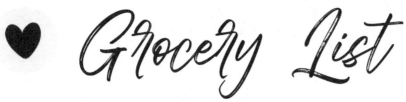

Grocery List

PRODUCE

GROCERY BUDGET:

BREADS · PASTA · GRAINS

DAIRY · CHEESE · EGGS

MEAT · POULTRY · FISH

SNACKS · BEVERAGES

CANNED · FROZEN

NON-FOOD ITEMS

notes

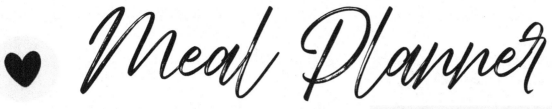

Meal Planner

WEEK NUMBER:

MONDAY

TUESDAY

WEDNESDAY

THURSDAY

FRIDAY

SATURDAY

SUNDAY

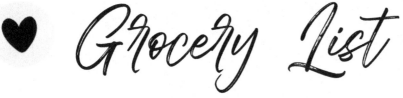

Grocery List

PRODUCE

BREADS • PASTA • GRAINS

MEAT • POULTRY • FISH

DAIRY • CHEESE • EGGS

CANNED • FROZEN

SNACKS • BEVERAGES

NON-FOOD ITEMS

notes

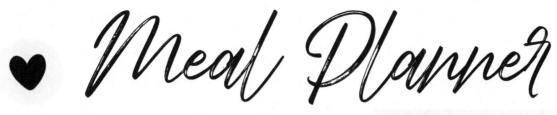

Meal Planner

WEEK NUMBER:

MONDAY

TUESDAY

WEDNESDAY

THURSDAY

FRIDAY

SATURDAY

SUNDAY

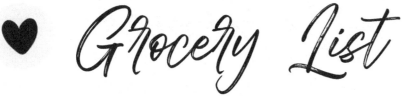

Grocery List

GROCERY BUDGET:

PRODUCE

BREADS · PASTA · GRAINS

MEAT · POULTRY · FISH

DAIRY · CHEESE · EGGS

CANNED · FROZEN

SNACKS · BEVERAGES

NON-FOOD ITEMS

notes

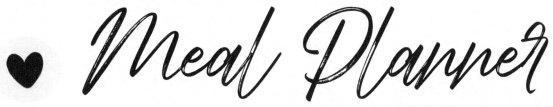

Meal Planner

WEEK NUMBER:

MONDAY

TUESDAY

WEDNESDAY

THURSDAY

FRIDAY

SATURDAY

SUNDAY

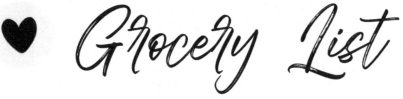

Grocery List

GROCERY BUDGET:

PRODUCE

BREADS · PASTA · GRAINS

MEAT · POULTRY · FISH

DAIRY · CHEESE · EGGS

SNACKS · BEVERAGES

CANNED · FROZEN

NON-FOOD ITEMS

notes

Notes

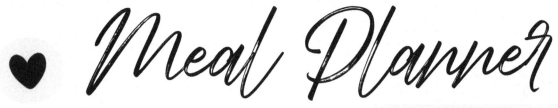

Meal Planner

WEEK NUMBER:

MONDAY

TUESDAY

WEDNESDAY

THURSDAY

FRIDAY

SATURDAY

SUNDAY

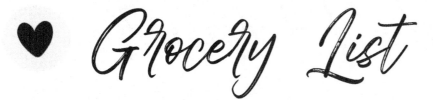

Grocery List

PRODUCE

GROCERY BUDGET:

BREADS · PASTA · GRAINS

MEAT · POULTRY · FISH

DAIRY · CHEESE · EGGS

SNACKS · BEVERAGES

CANNED · FROZEN

NON-FOOD ITEMS

notes

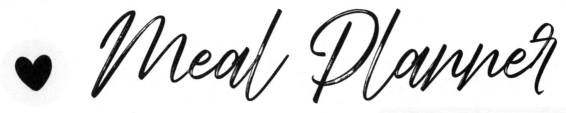

Meal Planner

WEEK NUMBER:

MONDAY

TUESDAY

WEDNESDAY

THURSDAY

FRIDAY

SATURDAY

SUNDAY

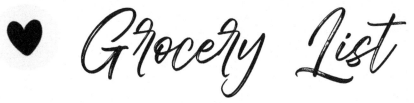

Grocery List

GROCERY BUDGET:

PRODUCE

MEAT · POULTRY · FISH

CANNED · FROZEN

BREADS · PASTA · GRAINS

DAIRY · CHEESE · EGGS

SNACKS · BEVERAGES

NON-FOOD ITEMS

notes

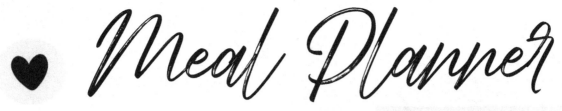

Meal Planner

WEEK NUMBER:

MONDAY

TUESDAY

WEDNESDAY

THURSDAY

FRIDAY

SATURDAY

SUNDAY

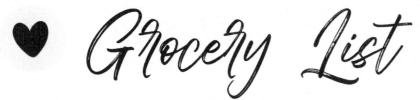

Grocery List

GROCERY BUDGET:

PRODUCE

BREADS • PASTA • GRAINS

MEAT • POULTRY • FISH

DAIRY • CHEESE • EGGS

CANNED • FROZEN

SNACKS • BEVERAGES

NON-FOOD ITEMS

notes

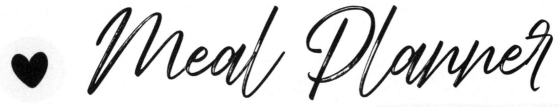 **Meal Planner**

WEEK NUMBER:

MONDAY

TUESDAY

WEDNESDAY

THURSDAY

FRIDAY

SATURDAY

SUNDAY

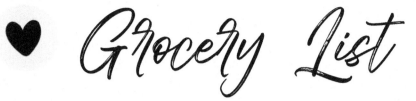

Grocery List

GROCERY BUDGET:

PRODUCE

_____
_____
_____
_____
_____
_____

BREADS · PASTA · GRAINS

_____
_____
_____
_____
_____
_____

MEAT · POULTRY · FISH

_____
_____
_____
_____
_____

DAIRY · CHEESE · EGGS

_____
_____
_____
_____
_____
_____

CANNED · FROZEN

_____
_____
_____
_____
_____

SNACKS · BEVERAGES

_____
_____
_____
_____
_____

NON-FOOD ITEMS

_____
_____
_____
_____

notes

Notes

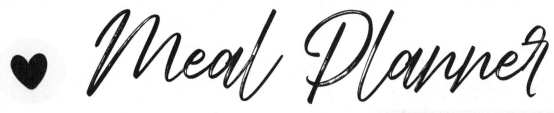

Meal Planner

WEEK NUMBER:

MONDAY

TUESDAY

WEDNESDAY

THURSDAY

FRIDAY

SATURDAY

SUNDAY

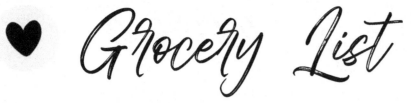

Grocery List

GROCERY BUDGET:

PRODUCE

BREADS · PASTA · GRAINS

DAIRY · CHEESE · EGGS

MEAT · POULTRY · FISH

SNACKS · BEVERAGES

CANNED · FROZEN

NON-FOOD ITEMS

notes

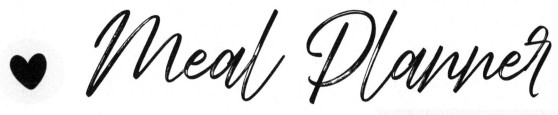

Meal Planner

WEEK NUMBER:

MONDAY

TUESDAY

WEDNESDAY

THURSDAY

FRIDAY

SATURDAY

SUNDAY

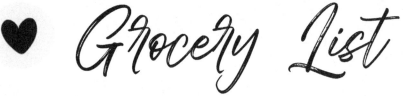

Grocery List

PRODUCE

BREADS · PASTA · GRAINS

MEAT · POULTRY · FISH

DAIRY · CHEESE · EGGS

SNACKS · BEVERAGES

CANNED · FROZEN

NON-FOOD ITEMS

notes

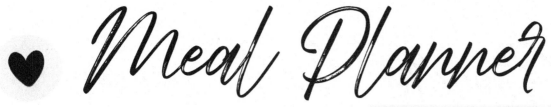

Meal Planner

WEEK NUMBER:

MONDAY

TUESDAY

WEDNESDAY

THURSDAY

FRIDAY

SATURDAY

SUNDAY

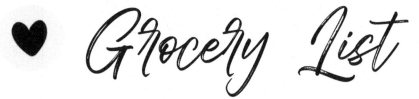

Grocery List

GROCERY BUDGET:

BREADS • PASTA • GRAINS

PRODUCE

MEAT • POULTRY • FISH

DAIRY • CHEESE • EGGS

SNACKS • BEVERAGES

CANNED • FROZEN

NON-FOOD ITEMS

notes

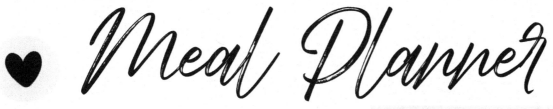

Meal Planner

WEEK NUMBER:

MONDAY

TUESDAY

WEDNESDAY

THURSDAY

FRIDAY

SATURDAY

SUNDAY

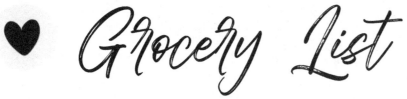

Grocery List

GROCERY BUDGET:

PRODUCE

_____
_____
_____
_____
_____
_____

MEAT • POULTRY • FISH

_____
_____
_____
_____
_____

CANNED • FROZEN

_____
_____
_____
_____
_____

BREADS • PASTA • GRAINS

_____
_____
_____
_____
_____

DAIRY • CHEESE • EGGS

_____
_____
_____
_____

SNACKS • BEVERAGES

_____
_____
_____
_____
_____

NON-FOOD ITEMS

_____
_____
_____
_____

notes

Notes

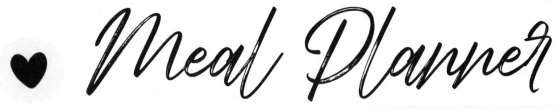

Meal Planner

WEEK NUMBER:

MONDAY

TUESDAY

WEDNESDAY

THURSDAY

FRIDAY

SATURDAY

SUNDAY

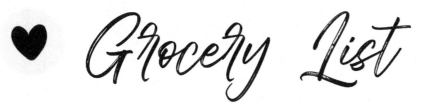

Grocery List

GROCERY BUDGET:

PRODUCE

_____
_____
_____
_____
_____
_____

MEAT · POULTRY · FISH

_____
_____
_____
_____
_____
_____

CANNED · FROZEN

_____
_____
_____
_____
_____
_____

BREADS · PASTA · GRAINS

_____
_____
_____
_____
_____

DAIRY · CHEESE · EGGS

_____
_____
_____
_____
_____
_____

SNACKS · BEVERAGES

_____
_____
_____
_____
_____

NON-FOOD ITEMS

_____
_____
_____
_____

notes

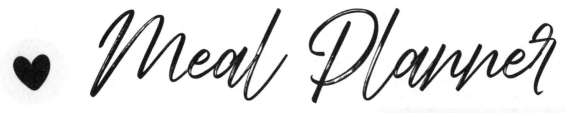

Meal Planner

WEEK NUMBER:

MONDAY

TUESDAY

WEDNESDAY

THURSDAY

FRIDAY

SATURDAY

SUNDAY

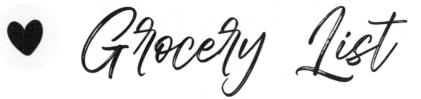

Grocery List

GROCERY BUDGET:

PRODUCE

MEAT • POULTRY • FISH

CANNED • FROZEN

notes

BREADS • PASTA • GRAINS

DAIRY • CHEESE • EGGS

SNACKS • BEVERAGES

NON-FOOD ITEMS

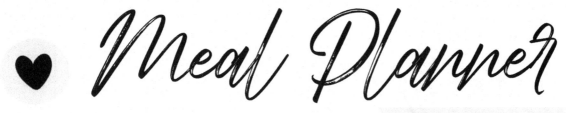

Meal Planner

WEEK NUMBER:

MONDAY

TUESDAY

WEDNESDAY

THURSDAY

FRIDAY

SATURDAY

SUNDAY

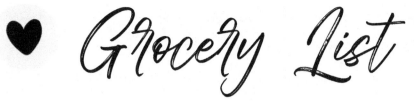

Grocery List

GROCERY BUDGET:

PRODUCE

_____
_____
_____
_____
_____
_____

MEAT · POULTRY · FISH

_____
_____
_____
_____
_____
_____

CANNED · FROZEN

_____
_____
_____
_____
_____

BREADS · PASTA · GRAINS

_____
_____
_____
_____
_____

DAIRY · CHEESE · EGGS

_____
_____
_____
_____
_____

SNACKS · BEVERAGES

_____
_____
_____
_____
_____
_____

NON-FOOD ITEMS

_____
_____
_____
_____
_____

notes

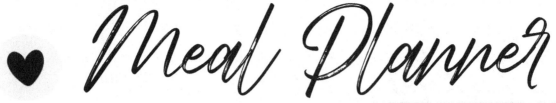

♥ Meal Planner

WEEK NUMBER:

MONDAY

TUESDAY

WEDNESDAY

THURSDAY

FRIDAY

SATURDAY

SUNDAY

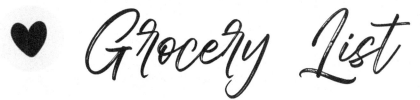

Grocery List

GROCERY BUDGET:

PRODUCE

BREADS · PASTA · GRAINS

MEAT · POULTRY · FISH

DAIRY · CHEESE · EGGS

SNACKS · BEVERAGES

CANNED · FROZEN

NON-FOOD ITEMS

notes

Notes

Notes

Notes

Made in the USA
Monee, IL
28 February 2022

92049676R00070